The Ultimate Guide To Dash Diet

The Only Book you need for Fast Natural Weight Loss, Better Health, Lower Blood pressure and Prevent diabetes including DASH Diet Recipes & Meal Plan

Elizabeth Grace

Table of Contents

Introduction — 10

Chapter 1. DASH to the Finish Line - Weight Loss and More — 14

Chapter 2. DASH Diet Project Phases — 16

    Phase 1: 14 Days to a Slimmer Waist — 16

    Phase 2: Re-Introduction of Sugar, Grains and Dairy — 23

Chapter 3. DASH Diet Breakfast Meals — 29

    Biscuit Recipes — 29

        Baked Turkey Sausage Cheesy Ciabatta — 29

Buttery Biscuits 30

Breakfast Cake Recipes 31

Sweet Breakfast Potato Cakes 31

Citrus Zucchini and Nutmeg Muffins 33

Whole Wheat Oat Pancakes with Low Calorie Maple Syrup 34

Quinoa and Spinach Pancakes 35

Milky Grits Waffle 37

Apple-Cinnamon Ricotta Muffins 38

Bran Cinnamon Cereal Muffins in Pineapple Bits 39

Bacon, Broccoli, and Egg Muffins   41

Egg Recipes   44

Quick Spinach Omelet and Pepper Relish   44

Dia de España Scrambled Eggs   45

Baked Eggs Southwestern Style   46

Shrimp-Artichoke Italian Omelet   47

Mini Turkey Sausage and Mushrooms Quiche   49

Goat Cheese, Bell Pepper, Oregano Frittata   50

Fruit Recipes   51

Baked Peaches with Peach Nectar Syrup 51

Strawberry French bread with Apricots and Cream Cheese   54

Grains   55

Breakfast Cinnamon Apples and Granola Bits   55

Baked Berry Almond Granola   57

Chapter 4. DASH Diet Hearty Lunch Recipes 59

Mediterranean Chicken Skewers in Low-Fat Yogurt and Curry   59

Smoked Turkey and Mango-Arugula Salad with Lime Dressing — 61

Cajun-Grilled Chicken with Mix Greens Salad — 63

Ranch Chicken Fajita Wraps — 65

Potatoes and Sausage Skillet — 67

Spicy Shrimp Moroccan with Pomegranate Sauce — 68

Tuna Salad on a Roll — 70

Classic English Tuna Melt Muffin — 70

Cheesy Asparagus and Tomato Primavera — 72

Asparagus Linguini Pasta — 73

Fettuccine with Asparagus — 74

Green Beans, Red Cabbage and Cheesy Gorgonzola Ziti — 75

Cold Sesame Peanut Spaghetti Salad — 76

Chapter 5. DASH Diet Delightful Dinner Dishes — 78

Thai Salad Steak — 78

Sirloin Steak Salad with Buttermilk Dressing — 79

Roasted Crusted Lamb in Merlot — 81

Pork Tenderloins with Mashed Cauliflower 83

Pork Tenderloins with Pear Maple Dressing 84

Beef Sirloin Plantain Kebab 85

Stir-Fry Beef with Broccoli and Ginger 87

Spicy Meatballs with Cilantro and Parsley 89

Chapter 6. DASH Diet Breads and Treats 91

Melt-in-Your-Mouth Apple Pie 91

Carrot Cake with Cream Cheese Frosting 92

Not-So Sinful Cinnamon Rolls 94

Cinnamon Granola with Berry Cheesecake Sweetness Yogurt 96

Overnighter Oats in Cherry Chia 97

Coconut Rosemary Nut-Free Bread 98

Grain Free Banana Cinnamon Bread 99

Coconut Cheesy Bread 100

Sweet Potato Bread 101

Chorizo Meatballs over Mashed Cauliflower 102

Conclusion 104

Introduction

I want to thank you and congratulate you for downloading the book, "Dash Diet: The Ultimate Guide To Dash Diet: The Only Book you need for Fast Natural Weight Loss, Better Health, Lower Blood pressure and Prevent diabetes including DASH Diet Recipes & Meal Plan".

This book contains proven steps and strategies on how to lose weight fast the natural way, lower blood pressure, and prevent diabetes.

Healthy weight loss management is the goal of all dieters. You may have thought that losing weight is usually done in the least period of time. At the end of your so-called crash diet, your weight rebound is definitely within a stone's throw away. This book can show you the proper way to lose weight – slowly but surely.

There were several studies that showed that this diet can reduce the risk of many illnesses, some of which are heart diseases, stroke and cancer. The DASH diet program, an acronym for is not a fad diet. It has been incorporated in hundreds of diet program for decades now. It is actually an acronym for Dietary Approaches to Stop Hypertension. So you see, it was developed as a complementary medical solution to those who are struggling with hypertension.

The core of the DASH diet revolves around achieving better health through a tested and proven weight loss program. This diet program encourages consumption of food that is rich in non-fat and low-fat dairy; vegetable, fruits beans and seeds. It is designed to reduce blood pressure by providing important nutrients like calcium, potassium and magnesium.

If you are among those who have a metabolic syndrome, hypertension or obesity then the DASH diet is for you. This book contains the information that you need to get started with this diet program. With this eBook, you can turn your life around. You will learn the ways to choose the right food to satisfy your cravings. You will be presented with customized recipes to help you lose weight without having to starve yourself or skip a meal. Why crash when you can DASH?

Thanks again for downloading this book. I hope you enjoy it!

☐ **Copyright 2015 by Elizabeth Grace - All rights reserved.**

This document is geared towards providing exact and reliable information in regards to the topic and issue covered. The publication is sold with the idea that the publisher is not required to render accounting, officially permitted, or otherwise, qualified services. If advice is necessary, legal or professional, a practiced individual in the profession should be ordered.

- From a Declaration of Principles which was accepted and approved equally by a Committee of the American Bar Association and a Committee of Publishers and Associations.

In no way is it legal to reproduce, duplicate, or transmit any part of this document in either electronic means or in printed format. Recording of this publication is strictly prohibited and any storage of this document is not allowed unless with written permission from the publisher. All rights reserved.

The information provided herein is stated to be truthful and consistent, in that any liability, in terms of inattention or otherwise, by any usage or abuse of any policies, processes, or directions contained within is the solitary and utter responsibility of the recipient reader. Under no circumstances will any legal responsibility or blame be held against the publisher for any reparation, damages, or monetary loss due to the information herein, either directly or indirectly.

Respective authors own all copyrights not held by the publisher.

The information herein is offered for informational purposes solely, and is universal as so. The presentation of the information is without contract or any type of guarantee assurance.

The trademarks that are used are without any consent, and the publication of the trademark is without permission or backing by the trademark owner. All trademarks and brands within this book are for clarifying purposes only and are the owned by the owners themselves, not affiliated with this document.

Chapter 1. DASH to the Finish Line - Weight Loss and More

To begin your DASH diet journey, you have to keep in mind that this is not a program for weight loss but rather, a way to enhance a healthier lifestyle. Keep in mind that this diet is low in cholesterol and fat. Here is a guide to help you get to understand what the DASH diet can do for you and your body.

Recommended Servings

The DASH diet does not support alcoholic or caffeinated beverages. It suggests that you take those in moderation (keep consumption to 1-2 servings a day).

More information on recommended servings:

Grains up to 8 servings
Vegetables up to 5 servings
Fruits up to 5 servings
Dairy products up to 3 servings
Poultry, fish and lean meat products can be up to 6 servings
Oils and Fat-based products up to 3 servings
Legumes, seeds and nuts up to 5 servings a week
Sweets or sugary products up to 5 servings a week

Steps to Success

No to Going Cold Turkey

The DASH diet does not force you to make a 360 degree turn on your eating habits. You should change your habits gradually and not shock your body and take the risk of bingeing on prohibited food in secret.

Job-Well-Done Treats and Diet Blunder Slips

Treat yourself to a non-food reward during the times when you have accomplished a day in the DASH diet. Non-food rewards are recommended since it teaches you the value that "Money can't buy Love" as the saying goes. Simple weight loss achievements can be rewarded with a spa treatment, haircut, new blouse you want or even a movie marathon with your friends.
Diet blunder slips should not be disregarded as well. Assess where you went wrong then start anew with what you have learned from it.

Let's Get Physical

The DASH diet supports the Low Blood Pressure campaign. Keep in mind to combine a healthy diet and an active lifestyle.

Chapter 2. DASH Diet Project Phases

Phase 1: 14 Days to a Slimmer Waist

For you to succeed in the first 14 days, you have to avoid whole grains and fruits for the meantime. The first phase is often the hardest but to you can hang on to craving bursts by eating low-fat dairy like low-fat yogurt or skim milk. No salt for this phase too since salt in your diet would mean water retention. Include leafy vegetables in your diet.

Help yourself to spinach, broccoli, cucumber, pepper or tomato. Do not think that the world has opened up and swallowed you whole for you can enjoy up to 6 ounces of meat a day. It is best that you combine a salad meal with fish, chicken or lean meat.

To survive Phase 1, keep these keywords by heart – low-starch, no grains, no fruits and no milk.

Day 1

Breakfast

Ham roll-ups with lettuce and tomatoes
1 slice of low-fat cheese
Plain yogurt
Tomato juice

Lunch

Turkey sandwich with tomatoes
½ cup carrots (steamed)
1 cup Sugar-free gelatin

Dinner

Baked Chicken (white meat)
½ cup green beans
1 cup mixed salad greens with balsamic vinegar dressing

Snacks (mid-day or before dinner)
1 cup plain yogurt

Day 2

Breakfast

Ham and Asparagus Quiche
1 cup of yogurt

Lunch

Turkey sandwich
1 cup baby carrots (steamed)
1 cup Sugar-free gelatin

Dinner

Pan-seared fish in olive oil
Asparagus (steamed)

Snacks (mid-day or before dinner)

2 slices of cheese
1 cup cherry tomatoes
1 cup Sugar-free gelatin

Day 3

Breakfast

1 cup Hot Cocoa with skim milk
2 hard-boiled eggs

Lunch

Whole wheat Turkey sandwich with tomatoes, lettuce and mustard
Coleslaw
Sugar-free gelatin

Dinner

Meat sauce in Squash pasta
Mixed greens in Italian dressing
Sugar-free chocolate bar

Snacks (mid-day or before dinner)

10 pieces unsalted cashews

Day 4

Breakfast

1 piece whole wheat bread
Scrambled eggs

Lunch

3 pieces of hard cheese
Roast beef in pita bread
Sugar-free gelatin

Dinner

Lasagna with Zucchini
Mixed greens in Italian dressing

Snacks (mid-day or before dinner)

10 pieces of Almonds
1 cup Sugar-free gelatin

Day 5

Breakfast

1 Omelet with green bell peppers and cayenne pepper flakes
6 ounces tomato juice
1 piece of celery

Lunch

Deli Turkey Sandwich in whole wheat
1 cup coleslaw
1 cup Sugar-free gelatin

Dinner

Roast Turkey Pasta in olive oil and garlic
Mixed greens in Italian dressing

Snacks (mid-day or before dinner)

6 pieces grape tomatoes

Day 6

Breakfast

Bacon and Bell pepper Frittata
1 cup steamed broccoli

Lunch

Fresh salad greens and baked mushrooms in olive oil

Dinner

Turkey French bread sandwich with olives and tomatoes
Mixed greens in Italian dressing

Snacks (mid-day or before dinner)

1 cup low-calorie Chocolate milk drink

Day 7

Breakfast

1 bowl of Oatmeal in prunes and plums
I cup of Decaf coffee

Lunch

Lentils with Arugula and Thyme salad with tomato salad in vinaigrette dressing

Dinner

Tuna and Tomato whole wheat spaghetti
Artichoke hearts salad with tomatoes in Italian dressing

Snacks (mid-day or before dinner)

¾ unsalted pretzels

Phase 2: Re-Introduction of Sugar, Grains and Dairy

You may call Phase 1 as "14 Days of Darkness" so rejoice and here is the light at the end of the tunnel. You can now re-introduce whole grains to your meals. These are the pasta, bread and cereals. You can have at least 6 servings of these ingredients in a day. Smile all you can since your favorite fruits are Phase 2's staple food. For your everyday diet, allot 5 servings a day of frozen or fresh fruits for they are your source of natural sugars. Dairy consumption is the same as Phase 1 – low-calorie, low-fat, skim, fat-free.

Here is a 7-Day Phase 2 DASH diet sampler. You may also find the recipes in these pages for your immediate reference.

Day 1

Breakfast

Hot Chocolate drink
Mini Turkey Sausage and Mushrooms Quiche
1 cup of Almonds

Lunch

Fettuccine with Asparagus
Sliced Bell Peppers
1 cup Sugar-free gelatin

Dinner

Beef Sirloin Plantain Kebab
Romaine Lettuce with Italian Dressing

Snacks (mid-day or before dinner)

Baked Berry Almond Granola

Day 2

Breakfast

Hot Chocolate drink
Shrimp-Artichoke Italian Omelet

Lunch

Crusted Mozzarella Chicken Nuggets
1 cup of watermelon

Dinner

Stir-Fry Beef with Broccoli and Ginger
1 cup of melon and cantaloupe medley
Snacks (mid-day or before dinner)

Strawberry French bread with Apricots and Cream Cheese

Day 3

Breakfast

Hot Tea
Banana-Cashew and Almond Pancakes

Lunch

Cheesy Asparagus and Tomato Primavera
1 cup of pineapples

Dinner

Sirloin Steak Salad with Buttermilk Dressing
1 cup of grapes

Snacks (mid-day or before dinner)
2 granola bars
1 cup of Decaf coffee

Day 4

Breakfast

Hot Decaf Coffee

Honey-Crusted Banana Muffins

Lunch

Cold Sesame Peanut Spaghetti Salad
1 cup of pineapples

Dinner

Spicy Meatballs with Cilantro and Parsley
1 cup of strawberries

Snacks (mid-day or before dinner)

2 wedges of Monterey Jack cheese
1 cup of grapes

Day 5

Breakfast

Milk (fat-free)
Turkey Bacon in Whole Wheat Sandwich

Lunch

Tuna Salad on a Roll
1 cup of pineapples

Dinner

Pork Tenderloins with Mashed Cauliflower
1 cup of apricots

Snacks (mid-day or before dinner)

2 granola bars
1 cup of sugar-free fruit gelatin

Day 6

Breakfast

Hot chocolate drink
Grain Free Banana Cinnamon Bread

Lunch

Green Beans, Red Cabbage and Cheesy Gorgonzola Ziti
1 cup of grapes

Dinner

Pork Tenderloins with Mashed Cauliflower
1 cup of raisins

Snacks (mid-day or before dinner)

1 large banana
4 pieces of unsalted low-fat crackers

Day 7

Breakfast

Warm soymilk
Sweet Potato Bread

Lunch

Cajun-Grilled Chicken with Mix Greens Salad
1 cup of strawberries

Dinner

Pork Tenderloins with Pear Maple Dressing
1 small apple (diced)

Snacks (mid-day or before dinner)

1 large banana
10 pieces of almonds (unsalted)

Chapter 3. DASH Diet Breakfast Meals

Biscuit Recipes

Baked Turkey Sausage Cheesy Ciabatta

Ingredients

1 cup sharp cheddar cheese (reduced fat)
1 carton egg substitute
1/2 cup green onions
1 lb. turkey breakfast sausage
8 ounces Ciabatta bread
2 tablespoons fresh parsley
2 large eggs
1 and 1/4 cups fat-free milk
Cooking spray

Directions

- Preheat your oven to 400 degrees F.

- On a baking sheet, line the Ciabatta bread cubes in one layer and bake in the oven for 8 minutes.

- As soon as the bread cubes turn golden brown and toasted, remove from the oven and set aside to cool.

- In a skillet, coat the pan with cooking spray and add the sausages.

- Cook the turkey breakfast sausages for about 6 minutes before adding the beaten eggs, cheese, egg substitute and milk.

- Meanwhile, combine the egg mixture with the bread mixture you have earlier set aside.

- In a baking dish, coat it with cooking spray and refrigerate for about 8 hours.

- After eight hours, it is time to preheat your oven once more for 350 degrees F and bake the casserole for 50 minutes.

- Once it is ready, remove the baking dish from the oven and serve the Baked Turkey Sausage Cheesy Ciabatta with parsley.

Buttery Biscuits

Ingredients

1 carton plain low-fat yogurt
1 tablespoon baking powder
1 teaspoon honey
1/4 teaspoon baking soda
1 tablespoon all-purpose flour

1/4 cup stick of margarine (reduced-calorie)
2 cups all-purpose flour

Directions

- Preheat your oven to 425 degrees F.

- In a pastry blender, cut the margarine until it crumbles.

- In a medium-sized bowl, add the baking powder, baking soda and all-purpose flour.

- In the same bowl, add the honey, yogurt and mix with the flour mixture.

- On a flat surface, line it with parchment paper and dust it with flour.

- Place the batter and knead it 5 times until you can cut it with a biscuit cutter.

- Transfer the kneaded dough to a baking sheet and bake for 10 minutes.

- Serve the Buttery biscuits with a drizzle of honey.

Breakfast Cake Recipes

Sweet Breakfast Potato Cakes

Ingredients

1 teaspoon onion
1 large egg
1/8 teaspoon salt
Ground nutmeg
1/8 teaspoon pepper
1 lb. sweet potato
1/4 cup all-purpose flour
Cooking spray

Directions

- In a small bowl, combine peeled and shredded sweet potatoes, potatoes, all-purpose flour, pepper, salt, egg and nutmeg.

- In a large skillet, grease with cooking spray and add all the ingredients.

- Toss ingredients to coat the vegetables with the all-purpose flour and cook for about four minutes.

- Flatten the cooked sweet potatoes and constantly stir until golden brown.

- Serve on a plate and enjoy your Sweet Breakfast Potato Cakes!

Citrus Zucchini and Nutmeg Muffins

Ingredients

Cooking spray
2 teaspoons grated lemon rind
1 cup coarsely shredded zucchini
3/4 cup skim milk
2 cups all-purpose flour
1/2 cup sugar
1 tablespoon baking powder
1/4 teaspoon ground nutmeg
1 large egg

Directions

- Preheat your oven to 400 degrees F.

- In a medium-sized bowl, combine the sugar, nutmeg, all-purpose flour, lemon rind, and baking powder.

- After mixing the ingredients well, add in the oil, milk, whisked egg and zucchini then set aside.

- Grease a 12-cup muffin tray with cooking spray, pour the batter and bake in the oven for about 20 minutes.

- Once the muffins are done, remove them from the pan and serve the Citrus Zucchini and Nutmeg Muffins.

Whole Wheat Oat Pancakes with Low Calorie Maple Syrup

Ingredients

1/2 cup whole wheat flour
2/3 cup regular oats
1/4 cup egg substitute
1 tablespoon baking powder
1/2 cup all-purpose flour
3/4 cup maple-flavored syrup (low calorie)
1 cup fat-free milk
Cooking spray
1 1/2 tablespoons vegetable oil
1 tablespoon sugar (powdered)

Directions

- In the glass container of an electric blender, put oats, whole wheat flour, baking powder and all-purpose flour. Grind them together and set aside.

- In a medium-sized bowl, combine the egg substitute, oil and milk then add it to the glass container.

- Stir the ingredients until they are well incorporated.

- On a hot griddle, grease it way cooking spray and pour in the hotcake batter.

- Cook until bubbles have appeared on top and flip to the other side.

- Once the pancakes are done, serve them on a plate and dust it with powdered sugar and drizzle low calorie maple syrup.

- Enjoy your homemade Whole Wheat Oat Pancakes with Low Calorie Maple Syrup and garnish it wish fresh fruits.

Quinoa and Spinach Pancakes

Ingredients

3/4 cup quinoa
1/4 teaspoon ground pepper
6 cups baby spinach leaves
1 cup salsa
1/2 teaspoon dried basil
4 teaspoons olive oil (extra-virgin)
2 garlic cloves
2 large eggs (whites only)
1/2 cup Parmesan cheese
1 and 1/2 cups water

Directions

- Preheat your oven to 350 degrees F.

- In a saucepan, boil water and when it is ready, add the garlic and quinoa.

- Cover the saucepan and simmer the quinoa mixture for about 10 minutes.

- After 10 minutes, uncover the saucepan and cook for another 2 minutes until the liquid is fully absorbed by the quinoa.

- In a large bowl, transfer the cooked quinoa and set aside to cool.

- Meanwhile, stir the egg whites in a small bowl together with the pepper, basil and parmesan cheese then pour into the large bowl.

- To cook the quinoa pancake batter, prepare another skillet and grease it will oil.

- Pour the batter in a skillet and cook each side for 2 minutes.

- In a baking sheet, grease it with oil and pour the quinoa batter then bake it in the oven for about 5 minutes.

- After 5 minutes, your pancakes are ready to be served on a plate and paired with salsa and spinach leaves.

Milky Grits Waffle

Ingredients

2 large eggs
3/4 cup buttermilk
Cooking spray
1/2 teaspoon baking soda
1/2 cup regular grits (uncooked)
1 and 1/4 cups all-purpose flour
2 teaspoons baking powder
1 tablespoon sugar
6 tablespoons butter (unsalted)

Directions

- Preheat your waffle iron and grease it with cooking spray.

- In a medium-sized saucepan, pour 2 cups of water and grits then bring it to a boil for about 15 minutes.

- When the grits have softened, add butter, baking soda, flour, baking powder, eggs and buttermilk.

- Once the batter is smoothly combined, pour 1/3 cup worth on the waffle iron and cook until golden brown.

- Once done, remove from the waffle iron and serve the Milky Grits Waffle with honey.

Apple-Cinnamon Ricotta Muffins

Ingredients

1 tablespoon baking powder
2 teaspoons ground cinnamon
1/3 cup light ricotta cheese
2 and 1/3 cups all-purpose flour
1 tablespoon vanilla extract
1 teaspoon baking soda
1 cup low-fat buttermilk
3 tablespoons sugar
3 tablespoons vegetable oil
Cooking spray
1 large egg
2 large egg whites
1 and 1/2 cups apple
1 cup sugar
1/3 cup 2% low-fat milk
2 teaspoons ground cinnamon

Directions

- Preheat your oven to 400 degrees F.

- In a large bowl, combine the sugar, baking powder, all-purpose flour, shredded apple, baking soda and cinnamon.

- Add buttermilk, vanilla, cheese, egg whites vegetable oil, and egg.

- When the wet ingredients are mixed, combine it with the dry ingredients and stir until the mixture moistens.

- Prepare a muffin pan, grease with cooking spray and pour the batter.

- Coat the batter with cinnamon and sugar on top then bake in the oven for about 18 minutes.

- Once the muffins are done, remove them from the pan and serve the Apple-Cinnamon Ricotta Muffins.

Bran Cinnamon Cereal Muffins in Pineapple Bits

Ingredients

1 can crushed pineapple
3/4 cup milk (fat-free)
1 cup shredded carrot
1 teaspoon ground cinnamon
1 cup wheat bran flakes cereal
1 teaspoon baking soda
1 and 3/4 cups all-purpose flour
Cooking spray
2 tablespoons butter
2 tablespoons water
1/4 cup sugar
1 teaspoon baking powder
1 large egg

Directions

- Preheat your oven to 350 degrees F.

- Prepare the muffin tin cups by greasing it with cooking spray.

- In a large bowl, mix together the baking powder, all-purpose flour, cinnamon, baking soda and sugar.

- In a small bowl, combine the beaten egg, milk, cereals, crushed pineapples with juice and the butter; set it aside for five minutes.

- In a small saucepan, bring the carrots and water to a boil then remove when carrots soften.

- Drain the saucepan from water and set aside the carrots in a small plate.

- In a large bowl, add the cereal mixture, flour mixture and carrots then spoon them in muffin cups.

- Pop the muffin cups in the oven for 22 minutes until it turns golden brown.

- Once done, immediately remove the muffins and serve the Bran Cinnamon Cereal Muffins in Pineapple Bits then garnish with carrot shreds and cinnamon powder.

Bacon, Broccoli, and Egg Muffins

Ingredients

6 cooked bacon
1/2 cup broccoli
12 eggs
1 small bell pepper
1 small bunch of spinach
¼ cup sliced and diced mushrooms

Directions

- Heat the oven at 350 degrees F.
- Line muffin tins with grease
- In a skillet, add the bacon strips and cook it to a crisp.
- Once the bacon is done, chop into little pieces.
- Break 12 eggs and mix with the pepper, spinach and mushrooms.
- Add the broccoli and bacon.
- In a colander, rinse and drain the broccoli before cutting it into little pieces.
- Pour the egg mix into the muffin tin and baked for 25 minutes in the oven.

- When cooked, garnish the muffins with a few bacon slices and serve.

Honey-Crusted Banana Muffins

Ingredients

4 eggs
1 cup ripe bananas
1/2 cup maple syrup
1 teaspoon baking soda
1 teaspoon vanilla
1/2 cacao nibs
1/2 cup walnuts (chopped)
1/2 cup tapioca flour
1/2 cup coconut flour
1/2 cup melted butter

Directions

- Set the oven temperature to 350 degrees F.
- Line the tin muffins with parchment paper.
- Mix all the ingredients, equally dividing them into the standard tin muffins.
- Place the muffin pans in the oven and bake for twenty minutes.
- Once done, set aside to cool and store in the refrigerator before serving.

Banana-Cashew and Almond Pancakes

Ingredients

4 pieces bananas (ripe)
1/2 cup almond
2 tsp olive oil
4 pieces large organic eggs
½ cup cashew
Black pepper to taste
Cooked bacon (crispy)

Directions

- Combine mashed bananas and pre-beaten eggs in a large bowl.

- Add the cashews and almonds and mix well until smooth and creamy.

- Season the batter with black pepper.

- In a small skillet, add ¼ cup of the pancake batter and cook with olive oil.

- Cook the batter for two minutes until bubbles have formed.

- Flip each side until golden brown.

- Once done, top the Banana-Cashew and Almond Pancakes with crisp bacon slices.

Egg Recipes

Quick Spinach Omelet and Pepper Relish

Ingredients

8 eggs
2 cups spinach leaves
2 tablespoons chives
1 recipe Red Pepper Relish
Nonstick cooking spray
1/2 cup cheddar cheese
1/8 teaspoon cayenne pepper

Ingredients for the Red Pepper Relish

1 tablespoon cider vinegar
1/4 teaspoon black pepper
2 tablespoons green onion
2/3 cup red sweet pepper

Directions

- In a skillet, spray cooking oil and heat it.

- Meanwhile, combine the chives, egg and cayenne pepper then add them in the skillet.

- When the eggs are cooked, add the cheddar cheese, spinach and pepper relish.

- As soon as the spinach leaves have wilted, transfer the omelet into a plate and top with the pepper relish and enjoy your Quick Spinach Omelet and Pepper Relish.

Directions for the Red Pepper Relish

- Prepare a small bowl and add the green onion, red sweet pepper, ground black pepper and cider vinegar.

- Toss all the ingredients in a small bowl and set aside to use for topping.

Dia de España Scrambled Eggs

Ingredients

3/4 cup seeded tomato (diced)
1/4 cup green onions (sliced)
1/8 teaspoon black pepper
3 large eggs
1/4 cup fat-free milk
Cooking spray
1/4 cup green bell pepper (chopped)
1 1/2 cups egg substitute
1/8 teaspoon hot sauce

Directions

- In a large skillet with cooking spray and add the onions, bell peppers and tomatoes.

- When the vegetables become tender, remove the skillet from the heat and set it aside.

- In a large bowl, combine the egg substitute, milk, pepper, hot sauce and eggs.

- In a saucepan, add the egg mixture and cook it.

- Stir in the vegetables from the skillet and mix it with the eggs.

- When the eggs are already cooked, remove the saucepan from the heat and transfer the contents into a plate.

- Serve the Dia de España Scrambled Eggs and enjoy!

Baked Eggs Southwestern Style

Ingredients

3 egg whites
3/4 cup enchilada sauce (from a can)
1 can black beans
Hot pepper sauce
2 cloves garlic
1 cup shredded cheddar cheese
2 cans diced green chili
1/2 cup green onions
2 tablespoons all-purpose flour
1 tablespoon cilantro
1/2 cup milk

3 egg yolks
Bottled salsa
Sour cream

Directions

- Preheat your oven to 325 degrees F.

- Grease a baking dish with cooking spray and add the cheddar cheese, enchilada sauce, black beans, green onions, green chili peppers, garlic and a few drops of hot sauce.

- In a medium-sized bowl, whisk the eggs with an electric mixer until its tips curl then set aside.

- Prepare a large bowl and combine your whisked egg yolks and flour.
- In a baking dish, add into the egg yolk mixture the following ingredients like milk, cilantro and beaten egg whites.

- Pop the dish in the oven for 45 minutes and once the eggs are done, let it cool for 15 minutes.

- Serve the Baked Eggs Southwestern Style on a plate and add a side dish of salsa and sour cream.

Shrimp-Artichoke Italian Omelet

Ingredients

2 cups egg substitute
Cherry tomatoes
4 ounces frozen shelled shrimp
3 tablespoons Parmesan cheese
1/8 teaspoon garlic powder
Cooking spray
1/4 cup green onions
1/2 package frozen artichoke hearts
1/4 cup fat-free milk
1/8 teaspoon pepper
Parsley

Instructions

- Defrost the frozen shrimps, peel, cut into halves and pat them dry.

- Cook the artichoke hearts based on the directions on its package then cut them into quarters.

- In a small bowl, add the garlic powder, green onions, milk, egg substitute and pepper; set them aside.

- In a skillet, coat it with cooking spray and cook the shrimps for 3 minutes.

- In the same skillet, add the egg mixture and cook through until it is done.

- Turn the heat off and remove the skillet and add the artichokes, parmesan cheese and let the skillet cool for 4 minutes.

- Your Shrimp-Artichoke Italian Omelet is done and ready to be served with parsley and cherry tomatoes on the side.

Mini Turkey Sausage and Mushrooms Quiche

Ingredients

1 teaspoon olive oil (extra-virgin)
1 cup 1% milk
8 ounces turkey breakfast sausage
3 egg whites
1/4 cup scallions
8 ounces mushrooms
1/4 cup Swiss cheese
5 eggs
1 teaspoon ground pepper

Directions

- Preheat your oven to 325 degrees F.

- Generously coat a muffin tin with cooking spray and set aside.

- In a large skillet, cook the turkey sausages, without its casing, for 8 minutes then set aside in a medium bowl.

- Using the same skillet, add oil once more to cook the mushrooms for about 7 minutes.

- Once the mushrooms are cooked, mix them with the sausages then add in the pepper, grated cheese and, minced scallions.

- In a small bowl, add milk, egg whites and egg then evenly divide the egg mixture among the muffin tins.

- Add the sausage mixture into each of the greased tin cups and bake in the oven for about 25 minutes.

- Once the sausages have turned golden brown, remove it from the oven and let it cool for about 5 minutes before serving on a plate.

- Enjoy your Mini Turkey Sausage and Mushrooms Quiche and have a hearty breakfast!

Goat Cheese, Bell Pepper, Oregano Frittata

Ingredients

2 tablespoons olive oil (extra-virgin)
8 eggs
1/2 cup goat cheese (crumbled)
2 tablespoons oregano

1 cup red bell pepper (sliced)
1/4 teaspoon ground pepper
1 bunch scallions (sliced)

Directions

- Preheat your boiler and prepare a large skillet.

- In a medium-sized bowl, add pepper, whisked eggs and oregano.

- In the skillet, add the scallions and bell pepper and cook for 30 seconds until they wilt.

- Combine the egg mixture with the wilted vegetables for 3 minutes to create a frittata.

- Sprinkle cheese over the cooked frittata and broil it in the skillet for 3 minutes until they eggs fluff up.

- Allow the Goat Cheese, Bell Pepper and Oregano Frittata to rest for 3 minutes before you serve it on a plate.

Fruit Recipes

Baked Peaches with Peach Nectar Syrup

Ingredients

4 peaches, halved and pitted
1/2 cup dried tropical mixed fruit (such as Sunkist brand)
1/4 cup slivered almonds, toasted
2 tablespoons graham cracker crumbs
2 tablespoons brown sugar
1/4 teaspoon ground allspice
1 (12-ounce) can peach nectar
1/2 cup vanilla yogurt, divided

Directions

- Preheat your oven to 350 degrees F.

- On a chopping board, remove the skin of 4 peaches, discard the pit and dice them.

- In a medium-sized bowl, combine the dried fruits, peach pulps, toasted almonds, brown sugar, cracker crumbs and allspice.

- In a baking dish, pour the peach nectar and mix it with the peach mixture.

- Bake it for 40 minutes until the peaches soften.

- Once the peaches are done, pour the remaining peach nectar from the baking dish.

- Serve and enjoy your Baked Peaches with Peach Nectar syrup and top it with a dollop of vanilla yogurt.

Berry Breakfast Summer Compote

Ingredients

2 peaches
1 1/2 cups blackberries
2 tablespoons white wine vinegar
2 cups fresh blueberries
1 and 1/2 cups raspberries
1/2 cup brown sugar
2 tablespoons lemon juice
1/2 teaspoon lemon rind

Directions

- In a saucepan, combine the grated lemon rind, fresh lemon juice, white wine vinegar, brown sugar and fresh blueberries.

- Cover the saucepan and simmer for 20 minutes then cool at room temperature.

- Prepare 6 small bowls and pour the blueberry mixture.

- Serve the Berry Breakfast Summer Compote with fresh blackberries, raspberries, and extra peaches on the side.

Strawberry French bread with Apricots and Cream Cheese

Ingredients

1 egg
1/8 teaspoon apple pie spice
2 egg whites
1/2 cup fat-free cream cheese
1/2 teaspoon vanilla
8 slices French bread
3/4 cup fat-free milk
2 tablespoons apricot spreadable fruit
1/2 cup strawberry
Nonstick cooking spray

Directions

- Coat a griddle with cooking spray.

- In a small bowl, combine the apricot spreadable fruit and cream cheese.

- Cut the bread in the middle and fill it with the cream cheese mixture.

- In a separate bowl, mix the vanilla, milk, egg whites, apple pie spice and egg.

- Dip the bread in the egg mixture, place the bread on the griddle and cook it for 3 minutes until golden brown.

- In small saucepan, place the remaining apricot spreadable fruit and stir it until it melts.

- Serve the Strawberry French bread with Apricots and Cream Cheese.

Apricots and Nectarines Casserole

Ingredients

2 tablespoons orange liqueur
1 cup Almond Fruit Granola
1/2 cup fresh blueberries
4 medium nectarines
2 tablespoons brown sugar
1 cup Almond Fruit Granola

Directions

- Preheat your oven to 450 degrees F.

- In a medium bowl, mix together the blueberries, orange liqueur and nectarines.

- In a casserole, add in the sliced fruits, add the brown sugar and pop the casserole in the oven for 8 minutes until the fruits are tender.
- Serve on a plate then enjoy the sweet and succulent Apricots and Nectarines Casserole treat.

Grains

Breakfast Cinnamon Apples and Granola Bits

Ingredients

1 teaspoon lemon peel
1/4 teaspoon ground ginger
2 medium apples
Ground cinnamon
1 tablespoon brown sugar
1 6-ounce container fat-free plain yogurt
1 tablespoon butter
4 teaspoons honey
1/4 cup low-fat granola

Directions

- In a large skillet, heat butter and add the apples. Cook for about 5 minutes until golden brown.

- Add ginger, brown sugar and cardamom with the apples and continue cooking.

- When the apples are tender, remove all the ingredients and transfer them into a plate and cool for 10 minutes.
- In a small bowl, mix the honey, lemon peel with the plain yogurt and drizzle over the apples and serve.

- You may garnish the Breakfast Cinnamon Apples with crumbled granola on top for a crunchy breakfast treat!

Spiced Walnuts and Apples Oatmeal

Ingredients

1 teaspoon ground cloves
1 cup chopped dried dates
2 tablespoons ground cinnamon
1 cup chopped walnuts
1 cup brown sugar
1 teaspoon ground turmeric
1 cup chopped dried apples
3 cups grain cereal flakes
1 tablespoon ground ginger
3 cups rolled oats

Direction

- In a large bowl, combine the dates, oats, cereal, walnuts, apples, brown sugar, cloves, turmeric and ginger.

- In a microwave, boil one cup of water and pour it over the large bowl.

- Stir the oatmeal mix and make sure every dry ingredient is softened and let it stand for 10 minutes before serving.

- Enjoy a filling Spiced Walnuts and Apples Oatmeal.

Baked Berry Almond Granola

Ingredients

¼ cup wheat germ (toasted)

¼ cup applesauce (unsweetened)
½ cup bran cereal
Cooking spray
2 tablespoons of almonds (sliced)
3 tablespoons of honey
Granola
1 and ¼ cup rolled oats
1/8 teaspoon ground cinnamon
¼ cup dried berries
1/8 cup cherries

Directions

- Preheat the oven to 325 degrees F.

- Prepare a baking pan, grease it with cooking spray and then set aside.

- In a medium-sized bowl, combine the bran cereal, toasted wheat germs, rolled oats, cinnamon, almonds, applesauce and honey.

- Mix all the ingredients together and pour them in the baking tray.

- Add the crumbled granola on top and bake in the oven for 25 minutes.

- Once the granola mixture is done, serve it on a plate and garnish with fresh cherries and dried berries on the side.

Chapter 4. DASH Diet Hearty Lunch Recipes

Mediterranean Chicken Skewers in Low-Fat Yogurt and Curry

Ingredients

1 medium yellow summer squash
1 large red sweet pepper
1/4 cup plain low-fat yogurt
1 teaspoon curry powder
1 tablespoon lemon juice
1/2 teaspoon red pepper (crushed)
1 teaspoon dry mustard
Soft pita breads
1 teaspoon ground cinnamon
1 pound chicken breast

Ingredients for the Tomato Relish

2 pieces large tomatoes
Ground pepper
1 clove garlic
1 teaspoon oregano
½ grape tomatoes
1 teaspoon thyme
1 teaspoon honey
1 tablespoon balsamic vinegar

Directions for the Tomato Relish

- In a medium-sized bowl, combine the halved grape tomatoes, chopped large tomatoes, balsamic vinegar, oregano, honey, minced garlic, fresh oregano, thyme and pepper.

- Cover the bowl and refrigerate for about 30 minutes and use as a side dish for the Mediterranean Chicken Skewers in Low-Fat Yogurt and Curry.

Directions

- In a zip-lock bag, add the chicken and place it in a bowl.

- Use another bowl and stir in the crushed red pepper, mustard, curry powder,

- lemon juice, cinnamon and yogurt.

- After mixing the ingredients, pour them in the zip-lock bag and shake to coat the chicken.

- Refrigerate the bag for 4 hours and set aside.

- Meanwhile, preheat your broiler and prepare six metal skewers.

- Once the marinade is done, insert the squash, pepper and chicken to the skewers and broil for 10 minutes.

- Wait until the chicken loses its pink color before serving with warm pita bread

- Preheat broiler. On 6 long metal skewers, thread chicken, sweet pepper, and squash, leaving 1/4 inch between pieces. Broil 4 to 5 inches from heat for 8 to 10 minutes or until chicken is no longer pink, turning once. If desired, serve with pita bread and tomato relish.

Smoked Turkey and Mango-Arugula Salad with Lime Dressing

Ingredients

1/4 cup fresh cilantro
1 cup smoked turkey
Lime Vinaigrette
4 cups salad greens
2 medium mangoes

Directions

- On a chopping board, peel and slice the ripe mangoes by about 1/8 of an inch.

- Prepare a bowl and add chopped turkey, cilantro; toss in the Arugula.

- Serve on a plate and drizzle Lime Vinaigrette on top.

Ingredients for the Lime Vinaigrette

1/4 teaspoon grated fresh ginger
2 tablespoons water
2 tablespoons lime juice
2 tablespoons peanut oil
¼ teaspoon Lime peel (shredded finely)
Roasted peanut oil

Directions for the Lime Vinaigrette

- In a glass jar container, mix all the ingredients together, cover the container and vigorously shake to incorporate all the flavors.

- Serve on a small dish as dressing for the salad.

Crusted Mozzarella Chicken Nuggets

Ingredients

1 cup almond flour
2 eggs
1/2 cup coconut oil
2 chicken breasts
onion powder
pepper
1/2 cup mozzarella cheese
Garlic powder

Directions

- Season the chicken nuggets with onion powder, garlic powder and pepper.

- Dip chicken nuggets into scrambled egg batter.

- In a separate plate, roll the nuggets on the cheese and almond flour mix.

- In a saucepan, prepare the chicken nuggets with coconut oil for 3 minutes until it turns golden brown.

- Serve right away and garnish with parsley.

Cajun-Grilled Chicken with Mix Greens Salad

Ingredients

1/2 teaspoon dried thyme
4 pieces chicken breast halves
1/4 cup cider vinegar
1/2 teaspoon cayenne pepper
1 and 1/4 teaspoons onion powder
2 teaspoons sugar
1 tablespoon water
4 tablespoon salad oil
1 medium carrot
1/4 teaspoon dry mustard
1 small red sweet pepper
1/2 teaspoon black pepper
1/4 teaspoon garlic powder

1 green onion
6 cups mixed salad greens

Ingredients for the Dressing

Salad oil
Cider vinegar
Mustard
Sugar
Water
Thyme
Onion powder
Garlic powder
Cayenne pepper

Directions for the Dressing

- In a glass jar, combine the salad oil, cider vinegar, mustard, sugar, water, thyme, onion powder, garlic powder and cayenne pepper.

- Shake the ingredients for the dressing and drizzle on the Cajun-Grilled Chicken with Mix Greens Salad

Directions for the salad

- Set your grill temperature to 170 degrees F.

- Combine the onion powder, salad oil, cayenne pepper and pepper.

- Brush the oil mixture on the chicken and grill for 15 minutes until cooked through.

- When the chicken is done, combine the mixed salad greens, green onion, red sweet pepper, and carrots in a large salad bowl.

- Add the chicken and pour the dressing before serving.

Ranch Chicken Fajita Wraps

Ingredients

1 small green sweet pepper
12 ounces chicken breast strips
1/3 cup cheddar cheese (reduced-fat)
1/4 teaspoon garlic powder
2 10-inch whole wheat tortillas
2 tablespoons ranch salad dressing (reduced-calorie)
Cooking spray
1/2 teaspoon chili powder
1/2 cup Fresh Salsa

Directions

- Preheat your oven to 350 degrees F.

- In a medium-sized skillet, spray cooking oil and add the chicken strips, garlic powder and chili powder.

- Cook the ingredients for about 6 minutes to remove the rawness of the chicken and to soften the sweet peppers.

- Once done, transfer the pepper and chicken to a plate and set aside.

- Line the tortillas in the oven for 10 minutes until it blisters and heats up.

- Remove when done and transfer to a plate.

- Get the chicken and red green peppers, sprinkle a handful of cheddar cheese and place it on the warm tortilla.

- Wrap the tortilla in a foil and place it back in the oven.

Ingredients for the Fresh Salsa Dip

1/4 cup green sweet pepper
1/4 cup red onion
2 tomatoes
1/2 teaspoon minced garlic
3 teaspoons cilantro
Black pepper
Hot pepper sauce (for added flavor)

Directions for the Fresh Salsa Dip

- In a medium bowl, add the minced red onions, tomatoes, garlic, cilantro and drop of hot sauce.

- Combine the ingredients together to make a salsa and chill for 30 minutes before serving.

- Serve the with Ranch Chicken Fajita Wraps and enjoy!

Potatoes and Sausage Skillet

Ingredients

3 to 4 tablespoons olive oil
1/2 pound smoked turkey sausage
2 medium onions
1 and 3/4 pounds red-skinned potatoes (unpeeled)
2 teaspoons cumin seed
1 teaspoon dried thyme
1/4 teaspoon pepper

Directions

- In a skillet, pour the olive oil and heat it together with the onions and potatoes for 12 minutes.

- Slice the sausages about ¼ of an inch and add to the potato mixture.

- Cook potatoes and sausages for 10 minutes until they become tender then add the pepper, cumin seeds and thyme.

- Serve on a plate and enjoy your Potatoes and Sausage Skillet!

Spicy Shrimp Moroccan with Pomegranate Sauce

Ingredients

1/4 cup fresh lemon juice
4 cups baby arugula
1/2 cup sugar
3/4 tsp. ground cumin
1/4 tsp. ground cinnamon
Cayenne powder
3/4 tsp. ground coriander
1 lb. large shrimp
1 and 1/2 Tbsp. olive oil

Ingredients for the Pomegranate Sauce

Pomegranates
Lemon juice
Sugar

Directions for the Pomegranate Sauce

- On a chopping board, cut the pomegranates in the middle and place the seeds in a juice reamer.

- Strain the juice and in a saucepan, combine the sugar and lemon juice with the pomegranate.

- Bring the contents to a boil and constantly stir to dissolve the sugar.

- Simmer and stir until the sauce thickens then pour them into a saucepot.

- Serve in a small sauce dish and pour on the Spicy Shrimp Moroccan.

Directions

- In a shallow pot, boil the lemon juice, sugar and pomegranate juice for 45 minutes.

- Heat a grill pan and shrimp and cook 2 then top it with arugula; remove and transfer to a medium-bowl.

- Now toss the cooked shrimp with coriander, cinnamon, cumin and olive oil then once the shrimp mixture is fully coated, toss in the arugula, olive oil and lemon juice.

- Transfer the shrimps and arugula on plate then serve with the Pomegranate Sauce.

Tuna Salad on a Roll

Ingredients

2 pieces Kaiser Rolls
Lemon juice
Black pepper
Lettuce leaves
1 can of tuna in olive oil
1 hard-boiled egg
8 tomato slices

Directions

- In a medium-sized bowl, combine the red wine vinegar, onions, olive oil and olive oil then marinate for about 5 minutes.

- Once it is fully marinated, add the tuna together with its oil and combine with more pepper, red wine vinegar and lemon juice.

- On a chopping board, cut the rolls in halves, add lettuce leaves, tomato slices, tuna salad and sliced eggs.

- Serve with pitted black olive on the side and enjoy the Tuna Salad on a Roll.

Classic English Tuna Melt Muffin

Ingredients

3 ounces Cheddar cheese (reduced-fat)
1/3 cup chopped celery
6 ounces white tuna in water
1/4 cup low fat Thousand Island dressing
Pepper
2 whole-wheat English muffins
1/4 cup chopped onion

Directions

- Preheat your broiler to prepare for this recipe.

- In a medium-sized bowl, combine the onions, salad dressing, celery and drained white tuna then season with pepper.

- In a baking sheet, line the halved muffins.

- Top each of the muffins with tuna and broil for about 3 minutes then top it with cheese.

- Place it back in the broiler to melt the cheese before serving the Classic English Tuna Melt Muffin.

Cheesy Asparagus and Tomato Primavera

Ingredients

12 small cherry tomatoes
3 carrots
1 sweet yellow pepper
1 sweet red pepper
2 tablespoons olive oil
1 bunch asparagus
2 tablespoons grated Parmesan
3 cloves garlic
1 pound penne pasta
1/4 teaspoon black pepper
2/3 cup half-and-half

Directions

- In a large pot, boil water and penne pasta.

- Once the pasta turns al dente, keep the water but transfer the pasta in a bowl.

- In a large skillet over medium to high heat, add garlic, carrots and oil then cook them for 4 minutes.

- Once the garlic is turning light brown, reduce the heat and add the asparagus; cook for 8 minutes.

- After 8 minutes, add in the half and half, cherry tomatoes and pepper.

- Stir in ¼ cup of pasta water you reserved earlier.

- Drain excess liquid from the pasta and transfer everything to a plate.

- Sprinkle freshly grated Parmesan cheese, toss the pasta once more time and serve it.

Asparagus Linguini Pasta

Ingredients

16 fresh asparagus
1 tablespoon olive oil
4 cloves garlic
6 medium plum tomatoes
1/4 cup dry white wine
1 tablespoon butter
1 package linguini pasta
1/4 cup fresh basil

Directions

- In a large skillet, add pepper and garlic then cook it with olive oil for 3 minutes.

- While the garlic is turning brown, set it aside and add wine and asparagus stalks.

- Cook the asparagus for a minute then add the butter.

- In a deep pot, boil water and linguini pasta for 5 minutes then drain when cooked al dente.

- Transfer the pasta to the large skillet and toss it with the asparagus; add torn basil on top.

- Once the pasta is fully coated with the asparagus mixture, serve it on a plate and enjoy a hearty lunch.

Fettuccine with Asparagus

Ingredients

9 ounces fettuccine
1 medium fennel bulb
1 tablespoon olive oil
1/2 pound fresh asparagus
3 medium tomatoes
2 ounces prosciutto ham
1/4 cup grated Parmesan cheese

Directions

- In a large saucepan, add salted water and pasta then boil it for 10 minutes.

- In a skillet, cook fennel and asparagus in olive oil for 2 minutes then add the drained pasta.

- Cook the pasta for 2 minutes before adding the prosciutto.

- Transfer the Prosciutto Linguini Pasta to a plate and sprinkle Parmesan cheese on top.

Green Beans, Red Cabbage and Cheesy Gorgonzola Ziti

Ingredients

4 cups spinach leaves
6 ounces ziti pasta
1/2 teaspoon dried tarragon
8 ounces fresh Italian green beans
1/2 cup crumbled Gorgonzola cheese
1/3 cup Italian dressing (fat-free)
1/2 teaspoon ground black pepper
1 cup red cabbage

Directions

- Add water, beans and ziti pasta in a large saucepan and boil for 10 minutes.

- Rinse the pasta and Italian green beans under running water, drain, and then set aside.

- In a large bowl, transfer the ziti pasta, Italian green beans, tarragon and radicchio and top it with gorgonzola cheese.

- Serve the Green Beans, Red Cabbage and Cheesy Gorgonzola Ziti on a bed of torn spinach and enjoy!

Cold Sesame Peanut Spaghetti Salad

Ingredients

2 pinches red pepper
2 teaspoons ginger
1 pound packed spaghetti
2 tablespoons light brown sugar
1/4 cup unsalted peanuts
4 tablespoons peanut oil
4 tablespoons creamy peanut butter
2 teaspoons sesame oil
1/4 cup green onion tops
2 tablespoons soy sauce

Directions

- In a medium-sized soup pot, add water and bring it to a boil for 8 minutes.

- Drain the pasta and transfer it to a large bowl.

- Add peanut out in order for the pasta to not stick with each other.

- In a small mixing bowl, add the ginger, peanut butter, brown sugar, red pepper and sesame oil.

- Pour the half of the sesame oil mixture on the pasta and toss it to evenly coat.

- Cover the pasta bowl with foil and refrigerate for 2 hours.

- Once chilled, serve the Cold Sesame Peanut Spaghetti Salad on a plate and top with chopped nuts and green onions.

Chapter 5. DASH Diet Delightful Dinner Dishes

Thai Salad Steak

Ingredients for the Salad

1 tablespoon vegetable oil
2 tablespoons soy sauce
1 medium carrot
1 pound London broil
1 clove garlic
1 bag coleslaw mix
1/2 teaspoon ginger
1/2 bunch green onions

Ingredients for the Dressing

1/4 cup white vinegar
2 tablespoons sugar
1 tablespoon vegetable oil
3/4 teaspoon grated ginger

Directions

- In a grill pan, cook the London broil for 12 minutes for a medium-rare doneness. Just keep in mind to flip the steak every 6 minutes for that.

- Meanwhile, in a zip-lock bag, mix the soy sauce, cooked London broil,

- vegetable oil, grated ginger and garlic then refrigerate for 3 hours.

- In a large bowl, combine the green onions, carrot and coleslaw mix.

- Prepare the dressing by combining the ginger, vegetable oil, sugar and white vinegar.

- Heat the ingredients in a small saucepan until the sugar melts.

- Toss the dressing into the salad and top with the steak.

- Serve the Thai Salad Steak on a plate and enjoy!

Sirloin Steak Salad with Buttermilk Dressing

Ingredients

8 cups mixed salad greens
1 recipe Buttermilk Dressing
1 medium yellow sweet pepper
1/4 cup fresh basil
8 ounces beef sirloin steak
2 medium carrots
1 cup cherry tomatoes
Cooking spray

Directions

- Grease a large skillet with oil and add the meat and basil.

- Cook the meat for about 3 minutes then remove the skillet from the heat.

- On a large serving plate, place the carrots, salad green, sweet pepper and tomatoes.

- Trim excess fat from the meat and slice them into thin strips.

- Serve the sirloin steak salad, pour buttermilk ranch dressing and garnish with sliced tomatoes.

Ingredients for the Low Calorie Buttermilk Dressing

2 tablespoons white-wine vinegar
1/4 cup mayonnaise reduced-fat
1/2 cup buttermilk
1/2 teaspoon salt (see note)
1/2 teaspoon garlic (granulated)
1/3 cup chopped fresh herbs (tarragon, chives, basil)
1/2 teaspoon pepper

Directions for the Low Calorie Buttermilk Dressing

- In a medium-sized bowl, combine mayonnaise, buttermilk, white wine vinegar, a little salt and pepper.

- Stir the ingredients until they become smooth.

- Note: The Dash Diet is a low-sodium, low-calorie food program. There is salt to be added in this recipe so you can omit it.

Roasted Crusted Lamb in Merlot

Ingredients

3 tablespoons dried cranberries
1 cup merlot
1/2 teaspoon nutmeg
2 cloves garlic
2 1-pound lamb rib roast
1 tablespoon fresh rosemary
3 tablespoons olive oil
1 tablespoon butter
1 tablespoon fresh rosemary
2 cups soft bread crumbs
1/2 teaspoon black pepper
1 tablespoon dried lavender

Directions

- Preheat your oven to 450 degrees F.

- On a chopping board, slice off the membrane and fat layers of lamb.

- Once done, prepare the marinade by placing the lamb roast, clove garlic, merlot and nutmeg in a zip-lock bag and place it in a baking dish.

- Refrigerate the lamb marinade for 4 hours.

- Meanwhile, in a skillet, heat oil and butter then add garlic and rosemary; cook for a minute.

- Once set, add soft bread crumbs, cranberries, pepper and cranberries in the skillet and mix well.

- After 4 hours, remove the baking dish from the refrigerator; serve the marinade juice in a bowl.

- Pat the lamb with the bread crumb mixture and line it on a roasting pan.

- Bake the lamb in the oven for about 30 minutes with a foil on top to prevent burning.

- Once done, allow to cool for 15 minutes before serving the Roasted Crusted Lamb in Merlot.

Pork Tenderloins with Mashed Cauliflower

Ingredients

1 cup Chicken Broth
2 pork tenderloins (trimmed fat)
1 can of organic mushrooms
2 Tbsp. Oregano
1 Tbsp. Basil
1 Tbsp. Garlic Powder
2 Bay Leaves
1 large can organic tomatoes (diced)

Ingredients for the Mashed Cauliflower

2 Tbsp. Butter
1 head Cauliflower

Directions for the Mashed Cauliflower

- Steam cauliflower, butter and pepper for 30 minutes and puree in blender.

- Serve the mashed cauliflower with Pork Tenderloin on a plate.

Directions

- In a crockpot, add pork tenderloin, diced tomatoes, mushrooms and spices.

- Lastly, pour the chicken broth and cook for 8 hours on low heat.

- Once the tenderloin is cooked, transfer to a plate and garnish with mushrooms.

Pork Tenderloins with Pear Maple Dressing

Ingredients

16 ounces pork tenderloin
½ teaspoon dried rosemary
1/4 teaspoon dried thyme
1/4 teaspoon black pepper
1 tablespoon olive oil
2 medium pears
1/4 cup maple syrup
2 tablespoons dried red cherries
2 tablespoons apple juice

Directions

- On a chopping board, place the pork tenderloins and trim off the excess fat then cut into thin slices.

- Prepare a large skillet, coat it with olive oil and cook the pork tenderloin for 3 minutes then remove and set aside.

- In a medium-sized bowl, mix together the pepper; thyme and rosemary then add the pork tenderloin.

- Use the same skillet to add the maple syrup, apple juice, dried cherries and pears.

- Bring all the ingredients to a boil to soften the pears.

- Once done, serve on a serving platter and garnish with slices of pear on the side.

Beef Sirloin Plantain Kebab

Ingredients

2 ripe plantains
1 tablespoon Taco seasoning
1 tablespoon cooking oil
12 ounces beef sirloin steak
1 medium red onion
2 tablespoons red wine vinegar

Directions

- Preheat your grill and spray cooking oil.

- Remove excess fat from the sirloin steak.

- In a small bowl, mix red wine, vinegar, taco seasoning, oil and steak.

- Toss the ingredients together to coat the meat and set aside.

- Take the skewers and thread the chunks of meat, onions and plantain.

- Brush the kebabs with olive oil and grill until the meat and vegetables are cooked.

- When you achieved the grill marks on the kebabs, serve them immediately with a side dish of yogurt dip.

Ingredients for the Yogurt Dip

1/2 cup plain yogurt
1/3 cup feta cheese
1 teaspoon lemon juice
1 garlic clove
1/2 teaspoon pepper
1/2 teaspoon hot pepper flakes
1/2 teaspoon dried mint

Directions for the Yogurt Dip

- In a food processor, add in the crumbled feta cheese, pepper, dried mint, lemon juice, plain yogurt, garlic clove, and pepper flakes.

- Set the processor to a pulse and blend the ingredients to achieve a smooth dip.

- Transfer the yogurt dip in a small bowl and serve with the Beef Sirloin Plantain Kebab.

Stir-Fry Beef with Broccoli and Ginger

Ingredients

8 ounces beef top round steak
1/2 cup beef broth (reduced-sodium)
3 tablespoons soy sauce (reduced-sodium)
2-1/2 teaspoons cornstarch
1 teaspoon sugar
1/2 teaspoon fresh ginger

Cooking spray

12 ounces fresh or frozen asparagus
1-1/2 cups sliced fresh mushrooms
1 cup small broccoli florets
4 green onions
2 teaspoons olive oil
2 cups cooked brown rice

Directions

- Start this recipe by trimming off excess fat from the round steak.

- Prepare the sauce by getting a small bowl to mix the cornstarch, soy sauce, sugar, ginger and beef broth.

- Set the first few ingredients aside and cook the vegetables.

- Coat a large skillet with cooking oil and add the mushrooms, green onions, broccoli florets and asparagus.

- Cook for about 5 minutes to soften the vegetables then once done, serve on a plate.

- In the same skillet, add the meat and olive oil; stir-fry the sliced round steak for 3 minutes, add the sauce and cook until done.

- Get the plate you set aside and add all the vegetables in the skillet.

- Cook for 2 minutes to heat the sauce.

- Serve the Stir-Fry Beef with Broccoli and Ginger on top of cooked rice.

Spicy Meatballs with Cilantro and Parsley

Ingredients for the Meatballs

1 egg
1 pound ground beef
1 small finely chopped onion
1/4 teaspoon ground ginger
2 tablespoons fresh cilantro (minced)
1 tablespoon paprika
3 tablespoons fresh parsley (minced)
2 tablespoons ground cumin
1/4 teaspoon cayenne pepper
1/2 teaspoon cinnamon
1/2 teaspoon pepper

Ingredients for the Sauce

1 cup of beef broth (organic)
2 tablespoons olive oil
2 cups crushed organic tomatoes
2 medium chopped onions
1/2 teaspoon black pepper
1/2 cup parsley (freshly chopped)
4 minced garlic cloves
2 teaspoons ground cumin
1/2 cup parsley (freshly chopped)
Pinch of cayenne

Directions

- In a large bowl, mix all meatball ingredients and roll them into large balls.

- Drizzle coconut oil and place the balls in a skillet pan and cook for 15 minutes until golden brown.

- Prepare a pot to cook the sauce and set heat to medium high.

- Add olive oil, garlic, pepper, onions, parsley, cayenne and cumin.

- Cook for about 10 minutes, then add the cooked meatballs and simmer for 15 minutes.

- Serve the spicy meatballs with sourdough bread on the side.

Chapter 6. DASH Diet Breads and Treats

Melt-in-Your-Mouth Apple Pie

Ingredients for the Apple Pie

1 egg white
1 pieces Pie dough (store-bought)
1 and 1/2 Tbsp. cornstarch
3/4 cup sugar
5 cups apples
1 Tbsp. lemon juice
1 tsp cinnamon
1 to 2 Tbsp. unsalted butter
1 pinch Nutmeg

Directions

- Preheat your oven to 450 degrees F.

- Line your table with parchment paper and roll out the pie dough.

- Once done, mold it on a pie plate and brush it with egg white; moisten the bottom with water.

- In a small bowl, mix the cornstarch, melted unsalted butter nutmeg then add to the pie plate.

- Add the apple slices and lemon juice.

- Cover the pie's crust with the other pie dough, brush melted butter on top and make 3 slits on top to allow steam to escape while baking.

- Turn down the oven's temperature to 350 degrees F now and pop in the pie plate and bake for an hour.

- Once the pie is done, prepare several plates and serve the Melt-in-Your-Mouth Apple Pie.

Carrot Cake with Cream Cheese Frosting

Ingredients

½ cup vegetable oil
2/3 cup fresh orange juice
2 tsp ground cinnamon
1 box yellow cake mix (plain)
4 large eggs
Flour (to dust pans)
1 box vanilla pudding mix
½ cup chopped walnuts
3 cups grated carrots
Vegetable shortening (to grease pans)
½ cup raisins

Ingredients for the Cream Cheese Frosting

3/4 cup chopped walnuts
3 ounces cream cheese, softened
2 and 1/2 cups confectioners' sugar
1 teaspoon orange zest
2 tablespoons fresh orange juice
2 tablespoons butter, softened

Directions for the Cream Cheese Frosting

- In a small bowl, use a hand-held mixer to beat the orange peel, confectioner's sugar, orange juice, cream cheese, and butter.

- On each cold cake, spread the frosting and sprinkle with toasted walnuts.

Directions

- Preheat your oven to 350 degrees F.

- Grease two round cake pans with vegetable shortening and dust them with flour.

- In a large bowl, use a hand-held mixer to mix the orange juice, cake mix, oil, cinnamon and eggs.

- Once the batter thickens, fold in the sliced carrots, nuts and raisins and transfer them to the pans.

- Pop the pans in the oven and bake for 35 minutes then remove from cake once done.

- Remove the cake from the pans and place one layer on top of the other then spread frosting on top and sides.

- Refrigerate the cakes for 20 minutes and once the frosting has hardened, slice and serve your hungry dessert lovers!

Not-So Sinful Cinnamon Rolls

Ingredients

1 tablespoon ground cinnamon
5 cups all-purpose flour
2 packages active plain dry yeast
1 teaspoon vanilla extract
2 and ½ cups water
2 cups light brown sugar
1/3 flour (for dusting)
2 tablespoons light corn syrup
1 package yellow plain cake mix
½ stick butter
2 sticks butter
½ cup granulated sugar
1 cup chopped pecans

Directions

- Preheat your oven for 350 degrees F.

- In a large mixing bowl, add water and yeast; stir until dissolved.

- Once done, mix cake mix, vanilla and 5 cups of flour.

- Cover the bowl and leave it at room temperature for 1 hour to allow the dough to rise.

- Meanwhile, in a saucepan, add the light brown sugar, pecans, corn syrup and 16 tbsp. of butter.

- After 1 hour, remove the cover from the bowl and give the cough a punch using your fist.

- Cut the dough in half with your hands and add knead it by a rolling pin.

- Cut the dough into pieces and roll into a big rectangular shape.

- Brush dough with melted butter and add cinnamon and sugar.

- You will create 15 slices when you cut the doll rolls and arrange them on a pan.

- Top the rolls with sugar, caramel syrup, and cinnamon mixture.

- Let the dough rise more for around 30 minutes before putting the pan in the oven for 32 minutes.

- Once baked, remove the pans from the oven and let it rest for 5 minutes.

- Serve the not-so sinful cinnamon rolls on a plate and enjoy!

Cinnamon Granola with Berry Cheesecake Sweetness Yogurt

Ingredients

1 container of Vanilla Greek Yogurt
1 pack of Whipped Cream Cheese
1 pack of Blueberries
A handful of Almonds
1 bar of Cinnamon Granola

Directions

- Whip cream cheese, vanilla Greek yogurt and crushed almonds in a bowl.

- Add a layer of cinnamon granola to a glass jar then add the yogurt mixture.

- Top with fresh blueberries, a dollop of the yogurt mixture and more cinnamon granola.

Overnighter Oats in Cherry Chia

Ingredients

1 cup of rolled oats (preferably gluten-free)
1½ cup of unsweetened almond milk
2 tablespoons of Chia seeds
2 tablespoons of pure Maple syrup
2 teaspoons of pure Vanilla extract
½ teaspoon of ground cinnamon
2 tablespoons of cocoa nibs (this is an option should you prefer this)
1 cup of raw Cherry Chia Jam
Chopped Cherries (for garnish)
Chopped almonds (for garnish)

Directions

- In a large bowl, add the wet and dry ingredients such as the rolled oats, Chia seeds, maple syrup, vanilla extract, unsweetened almond milk and cinnamon.

- Place the ingredients in an airtight container and refrigerate overnight.

- The following day, remove contents from the bowl and layer the oats and cherry Chia jam in 3 to 4 small jars.

- Garnish the tender and puffy oats with chopped cherries and almonds and serve immediately.

Coconut Rosemary Nut-Free Bread

Ingredients

1 teaspoon coarse sea salt
4 eggs
1/4 cup coconut milk
1/4 cup olive oil
1 teaspoon baking soda
1/3 cup flaxmeal
1 teaspoon freshly ground rosemary
3/4 cup coconut flour

Directions

- Preheat oven to 350 degrees F.
- In a bowl, beat eggs with a hand mixer.
- In a medium-sized bowl, add coconut milk, flax meal, baking soda, olive oil, sea salt and rosemary.
- Sift the coconut flour and add to the mixture.
- Add more coconut milk if mixture dries up, then bake for 45 minutes.
- Let it cool for 5 minutes before serving in slices.

Grain Free Banana Cinnamon Bread

Ingredients for the Bread

1 mashed ripe banana
1/2 tsp baking soda
1/4 cup coconut oil
2 eggs
1/4 tsp salt
1 1/4 cup almond flour
4 tbsp. honey
1/2 tsp vanilla extract
1/3 cup coconut flour
1 tsp cinnamon

Ingredients for the Topping

2 tbsp. coconut oil
2 tbsp. honey
1 tbsp. cinnamon

Directions

- Preheat oven to 350 degrees F.

- In a small bowl, add coconut oil, honey, mashed banana, and vanilla extract to the eggs.

- In a larger bowl, mix all dry and wet ingredients together.

- Grease a small baking pan with coconut oil and evenly distribute the mixture

- while adding the ingredients for the topping.

- Bake for 30 minutes until the bread's top is crunchy and golden brown.

- Serve immediately to enjoy.

Coconut Cheesy Bread

Ingredients

1/4 cup Romano cheese
2 cups Tapioca flour
1/4 cup coconut oil
1/4 cup coconut milk
2 eggs

Directions

- Preheat the oven to 450 degrees F.

- In a medium-sized bowl, mix dry and wet ingredients until well combined.

- If the dough is still wet, add another tablespoon of tapioca flour.

- Transfer to a cookie sheet to knead the dough.

- Once fully kneaded, brush coconut oil over the dough and sprinkle grated Romano cheese.

- Place the dough in the oven and bake for 15 minutes.

- Serve immediately with salad or beef stew.

Sweet Potato Bread

Ingredients

300 grams sweet potato flesh (roasted)
3 eggs
1 teaspoon baking soda
3 tablespoons coconut milk
Pinch of salt
1/2 cup coconut flour
½ piece of lemon (juiced)

Directions

- Preheat oven to 350 degrees Fahrenheit.

- Grease a small loaf tin and line with parchment paper.

- Set the food processor to pulse mode and fill with all the ingredients.

- Spoon the mixture in the tin and smoothen the top with a spoon.

- Transfer the tin pan in the oven and bake for 40 minutes.

- Open the oven hatch to cover the tin with foil then continue baking for 20 minutes.

- Once done, remove the tin pan and let it cool before serving in thick slices.

Chorizo Meatballs over Mashed Cauliflower

Ingredients

2 Tbsp. apple cider vinegar
1 head of cauliflower
2 lbs. Ground Pork
3 Tbsp. chipotle powder
1.5 Tbsp. paprika
1 Tbsp. onion powder
Salt and pepper
Chorizo Spice Blend
1 Tbsp. garlic powder
1.5 t black pepper
3 Tbsp. butter

Directions

- Mix all spices in a small bowl and set aside.

- Get ground pork then mix with spices and apple cider vinegar.

- Roll into 1-1.5 inch meatballs and place on the bottom of the crockpot.

- In a skillet on low heat, cook meatballs for 7 hours.

- For the Mashed Cauliflower, cut head of cauliflower and steam until tender.

- Place in food processor, add pepper, butter then puree until smooth.

- Plate the mashed cauliflower and meatballs with the drippings.

- Sprinkle with parsley for garnishing.

Conclusion

Thank you again for downloading this book!

I hope this book was able to help you to understand how you can have fast natural weight loss, better health, lower your blood pressure, and prevent diabetes.

The next step is to try the 2 Phase DASH diet program and cook up the recipes.

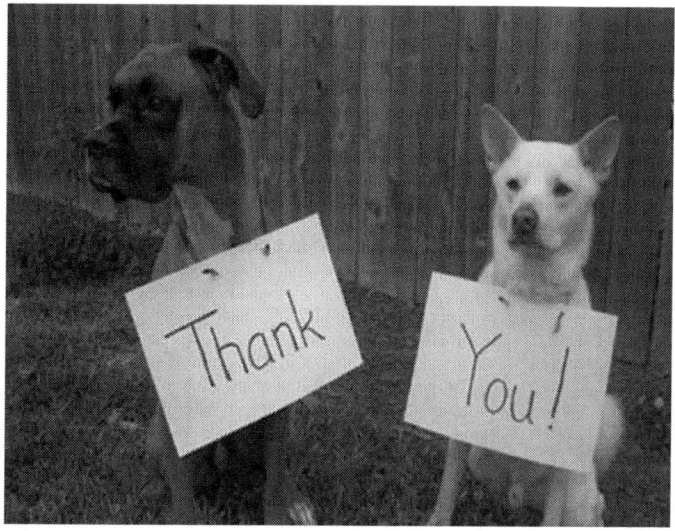

Finally, if you enjoyed this book, then I'd like to ask you for a favor, would you be kind enough to leave a review for this book on Amazon? It would be greatly appreciated!

If you liked this book, you may like these other books from Elizabeth Grace.

Check out more books from Elizabeth Grace.

http://www.amazon.com/Elizabeth-Grace/e/B00NCQPC5C

Thank you and good luck!

Made in the USA
Lexington, KY
30 October 2016